THE 14 DAYS METABOLISM MAKEOVER

A FAST TRACK TO WEIGHT LOSS, MORE ENERGY AND BETTER HEALTH

BRYAN K. KELLER

Copyright Page: © [2024] [Bryan K. Keller]

ISBN:

Published by: [Keith I. Hawkins]

Disclaimer: The information provided in this book is for educational and informational purposes only. The author and publisher are not liable for any losses or damages that may occur as a result of following the information presented in this book. Readers should consult with a qualified professional before making any significant changes to their lifestyle, health, or other aspects of their lives based on the content of this book.

2 |The 14 days metabolism makeover

Table of Contents

Chapter 1

The Metabolic Reset

1.0 Understanding Metabolism and Its Role in Weight Loss

Consider your body's metabolic rate as a mechanism that drives your body. It functions like a complicated, constantly functioning machine, processing the food you ingest and converting it into sufficient energy to power your daily tasks. Learning about your metabolism is essential for weight reduction and overall health.

The metabolism is made up of two basic procedures; that is, both anabolism and catabolism. The breakdown of protein converts nutrients and calories into smaller components, generating energy in the process. The term anabolism on the contrary hand uses this energy to build and restore tissues in the body.

A person's basal metabolism rate (BMR) represents the quantity of fats your body requires to carry out fundamental processes while you're asleep, which include inhaling and circulation of blood. Gender, chronological age, composition of the body, and genetics all impact your BMR. Knowing your BMR allows one to calculate the number of calories required to preserve, drop, or add bodyweight.

Learning about how your metabolism works is critical for successful weight reduction. In the event that you ingest a greater number of calories that your system requires, the additional energy turns up as fat, resulting in weight gain. On the other side, if you establish a deficit in calorie intake by eliminating a greater number of calories compared to what you ingest, your body uses stored fat as energy, and this leads to weight reduction.

Enhancing the rate of metabolism can help you lose weight. Consistent physical activity, particularly training for strength training, may assist you gain bulky muscles, and this eliminates more energy at resting than fatty tissue. A well-rounded meal plan packed with protein-rich foods, vegetables, fruits, and whole grains can also help to maintain a healthy metabolism.

It's crucial to realize that intense diets or excessive calorie restriction might decrease your metabolic rate, making it more difficult to reduce weight in the long term. Instead, focus on persistent lifestyle modifications like portion management, conscious food consumption, and frequent physical activity to promote an adequate metabolism and accomplish long-term loss of weight.

Furthermore, it is critical to remember that everybody's metabolic system is distinctive, and determinants including age, hormone changes, health issues, and degree of stress can all affect how effectively your body consumes and uses energy. This emphasizes the need of taking a comprehensive strategy to boosting your metabolism and attaining long-term weight loss.

Crash meals and extreme methods targeted at quick weight reduction may initially result in weight loss, but they frequently come at the expense of lowering your metabolism. This might lead to a pattern of weight loss and recuperate, referred to as yo-yo diets, which can have a severe influence on your metabolism in the long run.

As opposed to concentrating just on what's displayed on the scale, consider your entire physical and mental well-being. Pay attention to your body's signals for sensations of fullness and hunger signals, develop conscious eating by enjoying each meal, and strive for a nutritional regimen that includes a range of food categories to help your metabolism and general well-being.

Maintaining a lifestyle that includes consistent physical activity, proper water, decent rest, and managing your stress will help you improve your metabolism and burn calories more effectively. Making modest and lasting modifications to what you do every day can help you achieve and maintain a healthy weight in the long run.

Losing weight should be approached as an adventure of uncovering oneself and self-care, not as a fast fix. By learning about your body's specific demands and responses, you may develop a long-term and tailored strategy that corresponds with your objectives and ideals.

Understand that healthy weight reduction is more than simply losing pounds; it is also about enhancing your whole health and well-being. A healthy metabolism not only helps with weight loss but also supports your body's defenses, balance of hormones, and levels of energy.

Integrating diversity and moderation throughout your dietary intake, being well-hydrated, and paying attention to portion sizes may all help you maintain an optimal metabolic process. Furthermore, including frequent physical activity into your normal lifestyle, either by walking, strengthening exercises, or other types of exercise, will help you maintain your metabolism wellness as well as lose weight.

Finally, be nice to yourself during the entire procedure. Weight reduction experiences are susceptible to difficulties as well as successes, and improvement might not be as rapid as you would want. Celebrate minor triumphs, concentrate on the good changes you are implementing, and be compassionate with oneself as you journey toward achieving your goals.

In summary, developing an enjoyable connection with your own body and giving it the utmost respect and care it requires is more important than simply knowing numbers and calories when it comes to knowing the metabolism and its function in weight reduction. You can start on a revolutionary journey towards long-term weight loss, more energy, and general well-being by supporting a healthy metabolism with wholesome foods, exercise, and mindful lifestyle habits. Put your faith in the natural wisdom of your body, accept the journey, and acknowledge each step you take toward becoming a better, happier version of yourself.

1.1 Setting the Foundation for a 14-Day Transformation

Establishing the basis of a 14-day makeover entails establishing the framework for long-term adjustments that will help you achieve your weight loss and fitness objectives. Below is a full breakdown of how to lay the groundwork for an excellent 14-day improvement:

1. Set Unambiguous, achievable and Exact Targets throughout Your 14-Days Makeover. Either your goal is losing weight, gaining more energy, enhanced fitness, or overall wellness, having a clearknowledge about what you'd like to

accomplish can help you concentrate on your endeavors.

2. Evaluate Your Present Lifestyle: Consider your present behaviors, procedures, and lifestyles choices. Find areas from which you can make good adjustments to help you transform, which include dietary habits, sleep, physical activity, managing your stress, and self-care habits.

3. Plan: Establish a detailed plan explaining your actions over the 14-day timeframe. This plan should contain information about your nutritional modifications, workout regimen, hydration objectives, sleep pattern, and any other critical components related to the changes you are making.

4. Prioritize Nutrition: Start with filled with nutrients, healthy meals to support your change. Choose a well-rounded diet filled with vegetables, whole-grains, lean meats and beneficial fats to give your body the nutrition it requires to function properly.

5. Remain hydrated: Drink plenty of water through the day. Being adequately hydrated promotes metabolic processes, energy levels, and general wellness. Consider setting daily hydrated goals for making sure you're drinking enough water.

6. Exercise regularly to help your change: Consider pursuits which you love and are appropriate for your current state of fitness, such as taking walks, biking, aerobic muscular strengthening, or any other type of exercise that keeps you moving.

7. Obtain Enough Sleep: Emphasize adequate rest as a component of your change strategy. Strive for seven to nine hours of peaceful sleep every night to promote repaired cells, hormonal equilibrium, peak performance, and general well-being.

8. Maintain a good outlook and remain inspired for the 14-day change. To boost your mental health and resilience, engage in appreciation, graphical representation, declarations, and constructive self-talk practices.

15 |The 14 days metabolism makeover

9. Employ Assistance as well as Accountability: Enlist the help of associates, relatives, or a wellness coach to stay responsible and support you along your transition. Expressing your objectives with others may boost inspiration, accountability, and foster a feeling of belonging.

10. Measure Your Progress: Use a notebook or app to log your advancement, remark on your events, and celebrate your accomplishments during the 14-day change. Tracking your routines, actions, and accomplishments can help you remain on target and make any adjustments.

11. Organize your meals and light snacks advance in order to have nutritious alternatives accessible. Consider meal preparing on weekend or in batches to keep your eating habits consistent during the 14-day time frame.

12. Conscious Eating: Pay focus to hunger cues, relish each meal, and eat carefully. This might assist

you develop a healthy connection with food, avoid binge eating, and improve digestion.

13. Minimize Distress and Consider Caring for oneself: Employ stress-reduction techniques which include meditative practices, taking deep breaths, yoga, or getting outside. Employ self-love activities that encourage relaxation and mental health to help you change.

14. Remain Flexible and Respond to obstacles: Be prepared to change your strategy and accommodate to unanticipated obstacles during the 14-day transition. Remain adaptable, embrace setback with a development mentality, and prioritize development over excellence.

15. Recognize and appreciate tiny triumphs and progress made daily during the shift. Recognizing your accomplishments, no matter how minor, may increase your drive, assurance, and general feeling of success.

17 |The 14 days metabolism makeover

16. Evaluate and Learn: Consider your situations, lessons learned, and insights from the 14-day change. Consider what went well, what may be enhanced, and how to continue beneficial habits as well as modifications after the first period.

17. Establish long-term success Goals: Use the 14-day change to establish a long-term health and fitness objectives. Consider how you may maintain the good adjustments you've made, remain putting first your wellness, and build on your achievements for your future well-being.

18. Consider Expert Guidance: If anyone have special health problems or need individualized support, consult with a healthcare practitioner, a dietitian, or workout coach to guarantee a safe and effective 14-day change customized to your requirements.

Establishing a strong basis for your 14-day change with an achievable goal, a complete strategy, nutritious lifestyle choices, and an optimistic attitude creates a foundation for success in achieving your well-being and health objectives. Stay motivated, focused, and confident in your capacity to improve your life in 14 days.

Chapter 2

Kickstarting Your Metabolism

2.0 Metabolism-Boosting Foods and Nutrients

2.0.1 Metabolism- Boosting Foods

This is a full breakdown of metabolism-boosting nutrients and foods that help improve general health and metabolic processes function:

1. High in proteins foods: Proteins are needed for tissue repair and take more energy to breakdown than fats and carbs. To boost muscle development and metabolic rate, consume lean protein sources which include chicken, turkey, fish, tofu-based lentils, and low-fat dairy.

2. Fiber-Rich Foods: Fiber regulates digestion and keeps you satisfied for longer. Fiber-rich foods,

which include vegetables, as well as seedlings and nuts, can help enhance metabolism by promoting good digestion and taking in nutrients.

3. Green Teas: Green tea includes catechins, antioxidant that boosts metabolism and aid in weight loss. Drink a glass of green tea every day to enhance your metabolism.

4. Spicy Foods: Capsaicin, found in chili pepper and spicy sauces, can temporarily boost metabolism and burn calories. Including a little bit of spice in the food you consume may help boost your metabolism.

5. Whole Grains: Quinoa, brown grain, oats, as well as barley are high in dietary fiber and complex carbs, promoting energy and metabolic function. These meals assist to maintain blood sugar levels, avoiding energy dips that can decrease metabolism.

2.0.2 Metabolism-Boosting Nutrients

1. Vitamins B Complex: B vitamin aid in energy metabolism, converting food into useful energy for

the body. Whole grain foods, nuts, seeds, lentils, and leafy greens all contain B vitamins.

2. Iron: Iron helps carry oxygen and assist metabolism. To maintain appropriate iron levels, consume lean meats, poultry, shellfish, beans, and greens with dark leaves.

3. Omega three fatty acids Fatty Acids:Fatty fish such as salmon, mackerel and sardine fish as well as walnut and flaxseeds, include omega-3 fatty acids that boost metabolism function and calorie loss. These good fats also aid to decrease inflammation and improve heart health.

4. Magnesium:Magnesium plays a key role in approximately 300 biochemical activities in the body, such as energy metabolic processes. Magnesium-rich foods include nuts, seeds, green leafy vegetables, and whole grains, which can help with metabolism and energy generation.

5. Colorful vegetables and fruits contain antioxidants, which help reduce inflammation as

well as oxidative stress in the body. Antioxidants promote metabolic health by shielding cells from harm and may help enhance energy levels.

6. Probiotic-Rich Foods: Probiotics support a healthy gut micro biota, improving metabolism and general health. Consume fermented foods such as milk yogurt, kefir, sauerkraut, or and kimchi to promote gut wellness and metabolic function.

7. Avocado:Avocados include monounsaturated fats that boost metabolism and increase satiety. They also include critical minerals including vitamin E as well K, and foliate, and making them a healthy complement to any diet.

8. Berries are a superfood that boosts metabolism due to their high antioxidant, vitamin, and fiber content. Consume a variety of berries, including berries such as blue strawberries, raspberries, and blackberries, to promote general wellness and metabolism performance.

9. Nuts and Seed: Nuts and seeds include healthier fats, proteins, and important components that aid metabolism. Almonds, walnuts, seeds like chia, the ones from flax and pumpkin seeds among others are nutritional choices that can help improve energy and maintain a healthy metabolism.

10. Leafy Green Vegetables: Spinach, kale itself, Swiss the chard, and collard green are nutrient-dense and promote metabolic wellness. These foods are high in nutrients, vitamins, anti-oxidants, and dietary fiber, which make them an excellent complement to any metabolism-boosting diet.

11. Turmeric includes curcumin, a substance with anti-inflammatory and metabolism-boosting benefits. Including turmeric in your meals or drinking turmeric tea can assist improve metabolism health and general well-being.

12. Citrus Fruits: Oranges, lemons, grapefruit, and lime include vitamins C, anti-oxidants, and fiber. These fruits can aid with metabolism, immune

systems, and the breakdown of food, which makes them a great choice for general health.

13. Eggs: Eggs include high-quality protein, vital amino acidic substances, vitamins, and minerals. Eggs are a flexible and healthy food that can help with muscular building, metabolic processes, and satiety.

By include a range of metabolism-boosting nutrients and food items in your daily food intake, you may promote optimal metabolic function, energy generation, and overall well-being. To get the most out of these metabolism-boosting meals and minerals, be sure to eat a diverse and balanced diet, remain well-hydrated, exercise regularly, and promote a healthy way of life.

2.1 Daily Rituals to Rev up Your Metabolic Rate

This is a full description of daily practices that might boost your rate of metabolism and promote your general well-being and well-being:

1. Hydration: Start your day with a bottle of water to boost your metabolism. Staying hydrated is critical for proper metabolic processes and can aid digestion, nutrition absorption, and energy generation all through the day.

2. Consume a Balanced Breakfast: Feed your body with proteins, fiber, and wholesome fats. A balanced morning meal can boost your metabolism, normalize the state of your blood sugar, and give long-lasting energy to start your day.

3. Take Protein in Every Meal: Incorporating lean protein in every meal and snack helps promote muscle development and repair, increasing metabolic rate. Protein also has a larger thermic

impact, which means it takes greater amounts of energy to digest, hence assisting in calorie burning.

4. Maximize Strength Training: Add strength training activities to your exercise program to enhance muscle mass and metabolic rate. The connective tissue in muscles loses greater quantities of calories at repose than fatty tissue, therefore strength training is an efficient strategy to boost your metabolism.

5. Remain Active: Incorporate movement into your everyday routine, such as taking short walks, taking stairs instead of elevators, or indulging in active hobbies. Non-exercise activities thermogenesis (NEAT) can help to burn more calories and enhance metabolism.

6. Include HIIT or interval exercises in your fitness program. These strenuous activities can boost the rate of your metabolism, improve your cardiovascular health, and boost fat burning long after the session is finished.

7. Eat Consciously: Select high in nutrient snacks with healthy oils and fats, protein, and fiber to stay satiated and sustain energy levels. Limit sweet snacks and processed meals, as they can cause energy dumps and affect your metabolism.

8. Control Stress: Chronic stress can disturb hormone levels, including cortisol, which affect metabolism. Relaxation techniques such as meditation, yoga, and spending time in nature can all help to reduce stress and improve metabolic balance.

9. Obtain Enough Rest: Aim for 7-9 hour of quality sleep every night to promote metabolic wellness and a healthy lifestyle. Sleep deprivation can cause hormonal imbalances, boost appetites for unhealthy meals, and impair metabolism.

10. Develop Mindful Eating Habits: Pay close attention to hunger signs, slow down throughout meals, and enjoy your food. Eating with mindfulness can help you avoid overeating,

improve the breakdown of food, and achieve metabolic balance.

11. Minimize Processed Products and Sweetened Drinks: Limit the consumption of processed meals, sugary snacks, and beverages that can cause blood sugar spike and shuts down, adversely impacting metabolism over time.

12. Maintain Persistence and Patience: Remember that metabolic processes improvements take time, therefore consistency is essential. Focus on implementing these everyday practices into your everyday life, be patient with your progress, and have faith in your body's capacity to adapt and prosper with these beneficial habits.

13. Get enough water during the day to maintain hydration, the breakdown of food, and metabolic processes. Dehydration can impede metabolism, so have a water bottle available and drink regularly.

14. Consume Metabolic-Boosting Meals: Incorporate foods that promote metabolic processes into your diets and snacks. Green tea, spicy peppers, fruit and vegetables, nuts, seeds, and protein-rich foods can all help you burn more calories and maintain a healthy metabolism.

15. Spice up your dietary intake with metabolism-boosting spices such as spicy cayenne pepper, turmeric, ginger, and cinnamon. These spices can boost your metabolism, burn more calories, and add taste and diversity to your meals.

16. Thoughtful Movement: Practice meditation and yoga, tai chi, or stretching everyday to improve circulation, flexibility, and well-being. These mindfulness workouts can improve metabolism health and lower distress.

17. Spend Time Outside: Enjoy nature whenever possible. Spending time outside can help decrease stress, improve mood, and promote balanced

circadian cycles, among other factors which can benefit metabolism.

18. Target After a workout Nutrition: Refuel alongside a healthy breakfast or snack including protein and carbs to promote muscle repair and refill energy storage. Timing your post-workout meal can improve metabolism and muscle regeneration.

19. Employ Sensible Eating: Understand your body's feeling of fullness and hunger cues for optimal sustenance. Eating mindfully can help manage the amount of food consumed, improve metabolic balance, and develop a positive connection with food.

20. Practice Relaxation Techniques: Enjoy stress-reduction activities like deep breathing, meditation, and gentle stretching. Stress management is crucial for maintaining hormone-driven control and metabolic wellness.

21. Recognize and appreciate your accomplishments, big or little. Recognizing your accomplishments, being optimistic, and praising yourself for making an effort will help you stay motivated and on track with your metabolic journey.

22. Obtain Professional Guidance:If you have special health problems, dietary limitations, or fitness objectives, speak with a healthcare physician, certified nutritionist, or fitness expert for tailored advice and help in improving metabolic rate.

By implementing these everyday practices into your routine, you may create a favorable environment for increasing your metabolic rate, promoting optimum energy production, and improving your general state of health and wellness. Stay committed to your goals, stick to your routines, and believe in the transforming potential of these rituals to improve your metabolic health.

Chapter 3
Transformative Meal Plans

3.0 14-Day Meal Plan for Sustainable Weight Loss

Day 1:

Breakfast:Mashed eggs alongside spinach and tomato salsa, whole-wheat toast, a snack of mixed berries.

Lunch: Grilled-chicken breast, quinoa, and roasted veggies.

Snack: Greek yogurt drizzled with honey.

Dinner: a salmon bake with the asparagus and a salad.

Day 2:

Breakfast: Overnight oatmeal with milk made of almonds, chia seeds, and banana slices.

Lunch: Turkey and avocados wrap with carrots sticks.

Snack: A handful of nuts (such as almonds, walnuts, or cashews).

Dinner: Stir-fried tofu, broccoli, and brown rice.

On Day 3:

Breakfast: Made up a smoothie with cabbage, pineapple, and Greek yogurt.

Lunch: lentil soup and pure grain toast.

Snack: Cottage cheese and pineapple chunks.

Dinner recipe: Smoked shrimp skewer and quinoa tabbouleh salad.

Day 4:

Breakfast: Whole grain bread with avocado mashed up and poached eggs. A garnish of sliced strawberry.

Lunch: Grill salad of vegetables with mixed leaves, tomatoes with cherries, cucumbers, and balsamic vinaigrette.

Snack: Grain cake and almond butter for a snack.

Dinner: Baked chicken, roasted sweet potatoes, carrots, and green beans for dinner.

Day 5:

Breakfast: Chia seeds risotto with a variety of berries and sliced almonds. A modest handful of seed from pumpkin.

Lunch: Chickpea and garbanzo bean filled peppers, served with a side salad.

Snack: The carrot sticks and hummus.

Dinner: Turkey burgers, cabbage wraps, and grilled Brussels sprouts.

Day 6: Breakfast: Yoghurt cheese together with honey, oats, and chopped bananas, a small amount of mixed berries.

Lunch: Lobster thermidor, kale salad, and roasted veggies.

Snack: Cucumber slices with falafel sauce.

Dinner: Stir-fried bean curd, mixed veggies, and basmati rice.

Day 7:

Breakfast: Protein shakes including chartreuse, oat milk with banana, and powdered protein.
Sliced apple and almond butter

Lunch: Lentil salad alongside veggies, potato salad and lemon vinaigrette.

Snack: Greek yogurt topped with granola.

Dinner: Barbeque chicken alongside tahini plus boiled broccoli.

Day 8: Breakfast: Egg scramble with spinach sautéed and whole grain bread. A handful of mixed nuts.

Lunch: Stir-fry of turkey and vegetables served over brown rice.

Snack: Rice cake with avocado.

Dinner: Baked fish with sweet potatoes and asparagus.

On Day 9, breakfast consisted of oatmeal with banana slices and almond butter drizzling, mixed berries with Greek yogurt

Lunch: Grilled prawns and hummus salad

Snack: Carrot slices with tahini

Dinner: Baked chicken thighs, roasted Brussels sprouts, and quinoa.

On day 10, breakfast consisted of chia bean pudding with milk from almonds, fresh berries, and hemp seeds, handful of walnuts.

Lunch: Grilled veggie and tofu kebabs served with quinoa.

Snack: Hummus with sliced bell peppers.

Dinner: Baked fish, roasted asparagus, and wild rice.

Day 11:

Breakfast: A toast with avocado with scrambled egg and cherry tomatoes, A mixed berry side dish

Lunch: Chicken and black beans chili with blended green salad.

Snack: Cucumber slices with tahini sauce.

Dinner recipe: Turkey meatball with noodles made from zucchini and marinara sauce.

Day 12: Breakfast smoothie includes kale, pineapples, Greek yogurt, and protein powder, full-grain toast with almond butter.

Lunch: lentil soup and whole grain toast.

Snack: Cottage cheese and pineapple chunks.

Dinner includes stir-fried tempeh with broccoli, among others, peppers, onion, and brown rice.

Day 13:

Breakfast: Mashed egg with asparagus and tomatoes, Healthy whole-grain muffins with avocados spread

Lunch option: Grilled chicken Caesar salads with handmade dressings and whole meal croutons.

Snack: Greek yogurt drizzled with honey.

Dinner includes baked mahi-mahi, quinoa pilaf, and steamed green beans.

Day 14:

Breakfast: A protein-rich smoothie with leafy greens such berries, almonds milk, and protein powder. A handful of almonds.

Lunch: A wrap with turkey, avocado, lettuce, and tomato.

Snack: Carrot sticks and hummus.

Dinner: Grilled veggie stir-fry with brown rice and tofu.

Congratulations on finishing the 14-day eating plan for lasting weight reduction! By sticking to this schedule and eating nutritious, balanced meals, you'll be well on your way to losing weight and enhancing your general well-being. Remember to keep making conscious eating choices, being active, and paying attention to your body's sensations of fullness and hunger cues in order to sustain your success in the years to come.

Chapter 4

Power of Movement

4.0 Exercise and Metabolism: Strategies for Success

Exercising is essential for increasing metabolism and promoting weight reduction. The following are some comprehensive suggestions for success with exercising and metabolism.

1. Incorporating strength training into your fitness program is essential for increasing metabolism. Muscles burns far more energy at rest than fat, thus increasing muscular mass which may boost your starting metabolic rate. Strive towards 2-3 resistance-training sessions each week, with emphasis on key muscular groups such as legs, back, chest region, and core.

2. High-Intensity Intermittent Training provided (HIIT): HIIT exercises consist of shortened periods of intense activity separated by brief recovery

intervals. This sort of exercise is extremely good at improving metabolic rate and calorie consumption both before and after a workout. Include HIIT training once or twice a week for the best metabolic results.

3. Cardiovascular activity, such as jogging, swimming, bicycling, or aerobic exercise, can assist improve the cardiovascular system while also burning calories. Plan for no less than 150 minutes of moderately intense cardio or seventy-five minutes of vigorous-intensity cardiovascular exercise each week to help with weight reduction and metabolic health.

4. Keep Active All Daytime: In addition to scheduled workouts, try to keep busy throughout the day. Take brief walks, utilize the staircase rather than the elevator, or perform stretching activities. These little spurts of movement could assist with keeping your body's metabolism up.

5. Mixing up Your Exercises: To avoid plateaus and keep the metabolism going, modify your workouts

on a regular basis. To challenge your body, try new types of exercises and vary the intensity, length, and regularity of your exercise regimen and avoid adaptations.

6. Give Priority to Sleep and Recuperation:Adequate sleep and recovery are critical for metabolic health. Focus for 7 to 9 hours of excellent sleep every night to help your body's natural operations, including metabolic regulation. Allow your muscles to recuperate in between strenuous exercises to avoid injury and encourage muscular growth.

7. Hydrating and refuel appropriately: Drink enough water during the day to promote metabolic activity. Proper hydration is required for effective calorie burning. To maintain your energy and metabolism throughout exercises and throughout the day, nourish your own body with well-rounded foods rich in protein, complex carbohydrates, and healthy fats.

8. Measure Your Achievements: Keep note of your exercises, progress, and physical sensations. Consider utilizing a fitness notebook or app to chronicle your exercise habits, track your results, and alter your exercises as required to continue improving your body's metabolic rate and fitness.

9. Establish Realistic objectives: Whenever it comes to physical activity and metabolic processes, creating attainable objectives is critical for achieving lasting results. Breaking down your objectives into smaller, more doable steps and celebrate your accomplishments along the way. This might help you keep yourself inspired and on schedule with your exercise goals.

10. Mind-Body Connection: Practicing yoga, the Pilate's method, or meditation can strengthen your body-mind connection, decrease stress, and promote general well-being. Stress has an effect on metabolism, thus finding techniques for de-stressing and relaxing might be good for enhancing metabolic performance.

11. Responsibility and Supports: Think about working out alongside a buddy, enrolling in a fitness program, or contracting a fitness instructor to help you stay accountable and inspired. Getting an advocate can help you enjoy exercise and stay committed to your health objectives.

12. Listening to how you feel: Take notes to the manner in which your body reacts to exercise. If you feel unduly tired, sore, or in pain, you should relax and allows your body to recuperate. Excessive exertion might harm your metabolism and general well-being.

13. Commitment is vital: Regular physical activity is essential for keeping a healthy diet. On those occasions wherein you do not feel comfortable working out and try to get some physical exercise in, even if it's only a quick stroll or a moderate stretching session. Developing a consistent practice allows your body to adapt and enhance its metabolic processes over time.

14.Seek Expert Advice: If you're dealing with particular health problems, injuries, or are confused regarding how to best optimize your workout program for metabolism, consult with an expert in physical activity, such as an accredited personal trainer or certified fitness instructor. They can give you individualized guidance and assistance based on your specific needs.

By applying these tactics and including exercise into your daily routine, you may successfully enhance your metabolism, aid in weight reduction, while enhancing your general state of health and wellness. Remember that making little, regular modifications over time can result in big increases in your metabolic rate and fitness level.

4.1 High-Intensity Workouts for Maximum Results

High-Intensity Exercises, also referred to as HIIT (High-Intensity Intermittent Training), are highly efficient and successful workouts that consist of short periods of intensive exercise accompanied by brief rest or lower-intensity activities. High-Intensity Interval Training (HIIT) exercises are well-known for their potential to increase calorie burn, cardiovascular health, and metabolism. Here are the specifics of intense physical activity for maximum outcomes:

4.2 Benefits of HIIT Exercises:

1. Burn a greater number of calories over a shorter period of time than steady-state exercise.

2. Increases metabolism and allows you to burn calories even after you've finished your workout.

3. Increases blood circulation and anaerobic capability.

4. Can be adjusted to different exercise levels and readily tailored to individual needs.

5. Promotes fat reduction while keeping muscular mass.

6. Requires minimal to no equipment and may be completed anywhere.

4.3 Structure of an HIIT Exercise:

1. Warming up: Start with a 5-10 minutes warm-up to get your muscles and circulatory system ready for the tough exercise planned.

2. Time intervals: Move between high-intensity training and proactive recuperation or rests. For instance, imagine a 20-second period of all-out exertion with 10-second of unwinding, repeated for a certain number of times.

3. Select workouts that target individual muscle groups or integrate full-body motions for a complete workout.

4. Conclude with a 5-10 minutescool down that includes mild cardio and stretching exercises to help alleviate muscular pain.

4.4 A typical HIIT fitness routine is as follows:

1. A warm-up: Jogging in place as expected, arm circles, and leg swings for 5 minutes.

Intervals: Do every workout for forty seconds. This is followed by twenty seconds of rest. Repeat the circuit three to four times.

I. Jump squat.

Ii.Mountain hikers'

Iii.Burping exercises

Iv.High thighs.

V.Plank with shoulder touches.

2. Cooling downward: Walk or jog gently, static postures for 5-10 minutes.

I. To achieve the best results, prioritize quality over quantity by performing exercises with perfect form and intensity.

Ii.As your fitness improves, gradually boost the degree of exertion and length of your interval workouts.

Iii. Remain hydrated and pay attention to your body; rest as required and push yourself to your limits.

Iv. Incorporate several kinds of workouts to target various muscle groups while keeping the workout difficult.

V. Keep track of your progress by recording the intensity, length, and number of exercises done in each session.

Vi. Allow adequate rest time between HIIT workouts to avoid overtraining and injury.

By combining high-intensity exercises into your workout routine, you may get maximum calorie burn, metabolic increase, heart rate regulation, and general wellness.

Chapter 5
Mindful Eating Practices

5.0 Mindful Eating Techniques for Portion Control

Eating mindfully is a discipline in which you are totally active and focused to the feeling of eating. By implementing mindful eating strategies, you may enhance your connection with food, become more aware of feeling full and satisfied cues, and encourage healthy eating behaviors, such as portion management. Here are several ways for practicing mindful eating to assist with quantity control:

1. Awaken your senses

Before you take a mouthful, examine your food's sight, smell, and texture. Enjoying the visual and olfactory elements of your meal may improve your dining experience as well as making you more aware of portion proportions.

2. Slow down

Slow down and relish every bite. Chewing your meal completely and pausing in between bites permits your body to recognize sensations of feeling satisfied, which can help you avoid overeating. Place the dishes aside between bites to allow yourself to savor the aromas and texture of your food.

3. Listen to your body

Pay attention to your body's sense of fullness and hunger cues. Before eating, rate how hungry you are on a scale of 1 to 10. Begin snacking when you are reasonably hungry (about a 3-4) and quit when you are pleasantly full (around a 6-7). Avoid eating till you're excessively stuffed.

4. Control of Portion and Plate Size

To make a piece appear larger, use smaller dishes and plates. Studies indicate that when presented with greater amounts on larger plates, people typically eat more. You can fool your mind into thinking that a piece is larger by using smaller plates.

5. Prudent Portioning

According to your energy and nutritional demands, serve yourself the right amounts. Until you gain confidence in your ability to estimate portion sizes visually, measure portions by employing cups, scales and or visual indicators (such as a portion of protein the size of your fist, or a portion of carbohydrates the size of your palm).

6. Eating Without Distractions

Turn off the television, put away electrical appliances, and concentrate entirely on food. When you eat thoughtfully with no interruptions, you are more aware of what your body is telling you and can better control your portion sizes.

7. Practice Being Grateful

As you begin your meal, spend a minute to express thankfulness for the food that you will soon consume. Developing a sense of gratitude and awareness around meals might help you develop a healthy connection with food and avoid thoughtless eating too much.

8. Check-In During the Meal

Checking in with oneself during your meal to monitor your hunger and contentment levels. If you find you are becoming less hungry or nearing fullness, take a moment to assess whether you should continue eating or reserve the remaining food for later.

9. Reflect on Your Food Choices

After you've finished your dinner, take a time to think on your dining experience. Consider how the food affected you physically and emotionally. Consider if you ate out of being hungry, boredom, or practice, and then employ this insight to guide your future eating choices.

10. Meditation for Mindful Eating

Practice mindful mealtime meditations to increase your consciousness and sensitivity to your food. Take a few seconds before meal to take a breath deeply, show thanks for your food, and eat slowly, paying careful consideration to each bite.

11. Maintain a food notebook

Taking down the foods you eat as well as how you're feeling prior to and following meal can help you spot trends, motivations for eating excessively, and opportunities for growth. A food journal can help people become more conscious of their portion amounts and eating habits.

12. Employ Empathy and Non-Judgment

Practice eating mindfully with self-compassion and without judgment. If you consume too much or stray from your plan, be gentle to yourself and utilize these moments to learn and develop rather than criticize yourself. Cultivating a happy mentality can help with long-term behavior modification.

13. Request assistance and accountability
Discuss your conscious eating adventure with a close companion, relative, or healthcare provider. A supportive network may offer motivation, accountability, and new insights on your eating patterns.

14. Embrace mindful movement
Combine mindful eating habits with exercise like meditation, tai chi, yoga, or walking. Physical activity done carefully may strengthen your attachment to your body and increase general well-being.

15. Appreciate small successes
Recognize and appreciate successes in mindful eating, making aware decisions, and listening to your body's signs. Recognizing modest

accomplishments can boost confidence and drive to maintain a nutritious eating approach.

By adding these extra mindful eating strategies and recommendations, you may improve your ability to exercise portion control, make conscious food choices, and create a healthy and long-term connection with food. Recognize that eating mindfully is a process that requires tolerance, being aware of oneself and a dedication to putting your well-being first via mindful nutrition practices.

5.1 Overcoming Emotional Eating and Food Cravings

Controlling emotional eating and cravings for food need a holistic strategy that considers both psychological and physiological components of the practice. Here are some tips for managing and overcoming emotional eating behaviors and food hunger pangs:

1. Recognize Triggers: Recognize feelings, scenarios, or occurrences that cause your eating

emotionally or food cravings. Common causes include tension, boredom, depression, loneliness, and even happiness. Creating a food journal might help you detect patterns and particular triggers.

2.Find Other Coping Methods: Rather of resorting to food to deal with emotions, try physical activity, meditation, deep breathing techniques, journaling, speaking to a friend or a psychotherapist, or taking up a hobby. Emotional eating can be reduced by learning healthier strategies to regulate emotions.

3. Exercise Conscious Eating: The practice of mindful eating is observing the sensory knowledge of meals without passing criticism. Slow down, enjoy every mouthful, and pay close attention to sensations of fullness and hunger signs. By eating consciously, you may become more aware of your body's cues and distinguish between physical and emotional hunger.

4. Maintain Delicious Snacks on Hand: Keep nutritious, tasty snacks in the fridge and pantry so

you can grab them when you have a hankering. Choose entire foods including veggies, fruits, nuts, seeds, yogurt, and whole grain crackers. Having healthy alternatives readily available might assist to reduce impulsive intake of unhealthy meals.

5. Design wholesome meals: This include foods that are rich in nutrients including lean meats, whole grain foods, veggies and fruits, and healthy fats. Consuming well-rounded meals at regularly scheduled times can assist to regulate your glucose levels and curb desires for sweet or high-fat foods.

6. Stress Management: Learn how to effectively handle stress and lessen its effects on emotional eating. This might include meditation, deep breathing, yoga, or gradual muscular relaxation. Regular physical activity might assist to reduce stress and enhance mood.

7. Receive Adequate Sleep: Make sure you receive enough sleep every night, since sleep loss can affect hormone control and boost desires for foods that are

not nutritious. Strive for 7 to 9 hours of good sleep every night, and stick to a consistent sleep routine.

8. Get Support: If you're battling with emotional eating, don't be afraid to seek help from friends, family, or a therapist. Talking about your thoughts and getting support from others might help you get through challenging times without resorting to food for comfort.

9. Self-Compassion: As you deal with emotions and food cravings, remember to be nice to yourself. Accept that setbacks will happen along the route, and concentrate on development rather than perfection. Approach oneself with the same compassion and understanding that you would extend to a friend undergoing comparable circumstances.

10. Consider Expert Assistance if Necessary: If your emotional eating behavior is seriously affecting your standard of life or you are incapable to cope with it on yourself, then consider consulting

a certified nutritionist, a psychotherapist, or counselor who specializes in eating disorders or emotional health. They can offer individualized advice and assistance to help you build healthy coping techniques and accomplish your objectives.

Employing these tactics and making progressive lifestyle adjustments can help you manage and conquer eating disorders and food cravings, resulting in increased general wellness and a better connection with food.

Chapter 6
Metabolic Superfood

6.0 Foods That Naturally Increase Metabolism

1. Proteins-Rich Foods: Protein takes a greater amount of energy to digest than carbs or fats, which might briefly enhance metabolism due to the thermal impact of food (TEF). Protein-rich foods include lean meats (like chicken, turkey, and seafood), eggs, tempeh, tofu, and other legumes (such beans and lentil), tabbouleh, and mozzarella cheese.

2. Whole grains are high in complex carbs and fiber, which can help maintain stable blood sugar levels and prevent insulin spikes that can inhibit metabolism. Choose whole grains including oatmeal, chickpea, basmati rice, grain such as

barley bulgur grains, wheat-based pasta, and whole wheat bread.

3. Spicy foods contain chemicals such as capsaicin, which can temporarily enhance metabolism by increasing the temperature of the body and promoting the release of heat. Incorporate chili peppers, jalapenos, cayenne pepper, and spicy seasonings in your meals to boost metabolism.

4. Green tea contains antioxidants called catechins that have been demonstrated to enhance metabolism and fat oxidation. Drinking green tea on a daily basis, whether cold or hot, can help with weight loss and improve metabolic health.

5. Caffeine, a natural stimulant, can briefly enhance metabolism by activating the brain's sympathetic nervous system and encouraging adrenaline production. However, moderation is essential, since excessive caffeine use can result in jitteriness, sleeplessness, and elevated heart rate.

6. Water-Rich Meals: Being constantly hydrated is essential to sustaining an effective metabolism since dehydration slows down the process of metabolism. Cucumbers, celery stalks, tomatoes, lettuce, melons, oranges, and strawberries are high in water and may aid you stay hydrated and assist your metabolism

7. Leafy green vegetables, such as kale, spinach, Swiss the chard, and collard greens, are low in calories but abundant in nutrients including mineral content, vitamins, and antioxidants. Their high amount of fiber may help enhance thoughts of fullness and aid in weight management.

8. Fatty fish, including salmon, mackerel, sardine fish and trout, are high in fatty acids known as omega-3, which have been demonstrated to improve metabolic health and decrease inflammation Omega-3s may help increase fat burning and insulin sensitivity.

9. Berries, including blueberries, raspberries, strawberries, and blackberries, are high in

antioxidants, vitamins, and minerals, which promote general health and metabolism. Its high level of fiber can also help manage blood sugar and increase fullness.

10. Nuts and seeds are rich in nutrients high in beneficial fats, protein, and dietary fiber, which may assist in helping you stay full and content. Almonds, walnuts as well, chia seeds, the seeds of flax and pumpkin seeds, among others, are all good metabolic support foods.

Integrating these metabolism-boosting items into your dietary regimen, along with frequent physical activity and other good lifestyle practices, can help you maintain an appropriate metabolism and improve your general wellness.

6.1 Adding Superfood for Energy and Vitality

Superfood are meals that are high in minerals, vitamins, anti-oxidants, and other beneficial nutrients that can enhance energy levels, enhance general health, and promote vitality. Listed below are several great foods recognized for their energetic properties:

1. Chia seeds include a variety of nutrients, includes omega-3 fatty acids, fiber, protein, and antioxidants. They can aid to maintain energy levels and deliver a consistent flow of glucose into your blood stream, which makes them an excellent addition to fruit smoothies' yogurt, as well as cereal, and baked goods.

2. Quinoa: A gluten-free whole-grain cereal rich in protein, dietary fiber, minerals, and vitamins. It delivers a steady supply of calories and can help regulate the level of sugar in the blood, which makes it an ideal option for salads, stir-frying, or as a rice alternative.

3. Matcha is a powdered green tea that contains antioxidants such as catechins and caffeine. It gives a prolonged energy boost without the jittery affects

associated with coffee. Matcha can be consumed hot or cold, or added to fruit drinks, lattes, or baked products

4. Spirulina is a green-colored algae rich in protein, minerals, vitamins, and antioxidants. It can improve energy levels, immunological function, and detoxification. Spirulina powder can be added to smoothies, drinks, or energy bars to improve their nutritional value.

5. Acai Berries:These little, dark purple berries are high in antioxidants, notably anthocyanins. They can help fight oxidative stress, increase energy, and promote overall vitality. Acai berries are great in smoothies bowls, yogurt parfaits, and as a topping on cereals or salads

6. Cacao: Cacao, the unprocessed form of cocoa, is high in anti-oxidants, flavonoids, and magnesium. It can enhance mood, boost energy, and support cardiovascular health. Add raw cacao powders or

nibs to smoothies, breakfast, homemade vitality balls, or desserts.

7. Macadamia Nuts:These delicious and creamy nuts are high in beneficial fatty acids, vitamins, and minerals. They offer a steady supply of vital nutrients and can improve cognitive function and cardiovascular wellness. Macadamia nuts can be eaten alone or mixed into salads, cereal, or baked products.

8. Goji berries are little red berries rich in minerals, vitamins, and antioxidants. They can increase energy levels, immunological function, and general vigor. Goji berries can be eaten alone as a snack or mixed with trail mix, porridge, or smoothies.

9. Bees Pollen is a nutrient-dense material gathered by bees from blooming plants. It is abundant in proteins, minerals, antioxidants, and vitamins, making it an excellent energy source. For added nutrients, apply bee pollen on the surface of yogurt, cereal, or smoothie bowls.

10. Coconutcontains medium-chain triglycerides (MCTs), a form of healthful fat that can deliver rapid energy. Introduce coconut oil, milk from coconuts, shredded coconuts, or water from coconuts into your diet to increase energy and hydration.

Including these super foods in your diet can boost energy levels, improve general health, and encourage vitality. Include them in every meal and snack as part of a healthy diet for maximum energy and well-being

Chapter 7

Lifestyle Changes for Long-Term Health

7.0 Creating Habits for Lasting Wellness

Developing long-term wellness habits entails establishing stable lifestyle adjustments that promote mental, emotional, and physical health. Here are some tips to help you develop and maintain behaviors that promote overall wellness:

1. Clear Goals: Define clear, attainable goals that are consistent with your wellness vision. Clarity on your goals is vital for developing meaningful habits, whether they be to improve exercise, manage stress, or cultivate a healthier diet.

2. Start tiny: Divide your goals into digestible chunks and begin with tiny, attainable adjustments.

Developing new patterns of behavior takes time, so tackle one or two adjustments at a time to avoid overwhelm and enhance your chances of success.

3. Be Consistent: Establishing habits requires consistency. Decide to put your new habits into practice on a regular basis—ideally, every day or according to a set timetable. To make sure your wellness practices become a part of your everyday life, prioritize them, set routines, and set reminders.

4. Create a Support System: Be in the company of individuals who encourage you on your path to wellness and who have similar objectives. Having a support network of friends, family, or online communities can help with accountability, inspiration, and support.

5. Monitor Your Progress: To keep accountable and inspired, monitor your behaviors and advancement. Utilize a calendar, routine monitor app, or notepad to keep track of your everyday actions, recognize

your accomplishments, and pinpoint areas that need work.

6. Mindfulness and self-awareness can help you better comprehend your routines, thoughts, and emotions. Mindfulness techniques like meditation, deep breathing, and yoga can help you decrease stress, build resilience, and improve your general well-being.

7. Prioritize self-care habits that benefit your body, thoughts, and soul. This might involve getting adequate sleep, eating wholesome meals, exercise frequently, employing relaxation techniques, and doing things you like.

8. Be Versatile and Adaptive: Be willing to change your behaviors as needed to meet your changing requirements, preferences, and situations. Life may be unexpected, so adopt adaptability and learn to adjust your routines to different situations rather than discarding them entirely.

9. Applaud Your Achievements: Recognize and celebrate your accomplishments, no matter how minor. Acknowledging your accomplishments and triumphs may raise your confidence, promote beneficial behaviors, and inspire you to continue your wellness path

10. Be Kind to Yourself: Practice self-compassion, especially after failures or obstacles. Remember that developing long-term habits requires time and work, and it is OK to make mistakes along the way. As you strive toward your wellness objectives, be patient, empathetic, and encouraging with yourself.

By adopting these tactics into your daily routine, you may develop habits that promote long-term wellbeing and lead to a healthier, more enjoyable, and more meaningful living.

7.1 Stress Management and Sleep for Metabolic Balance

Long-term stress and insufficient sleep may interfere with the regulation of hormones, improve desire to eat, hinder digestion, and give rise to excessive weight develop and other health problems. To achieve metabolic balance, management of stress and sleep play critical roles.

7.1.1 Stress Management:

1. Hormonal Effects: Chronic stress causes the production of stress hormones such as cortisol, which can result in increased desire for food, hunger pangs for high-calorie meals, and belly fat storage. Increased levels of cortisol can also impair insulin sensitivity, leading to metabolic dysfunction.

2. Mindful Practices: Meditation, respiration exercises, yoga, and tai chi can all assist to decrease stress and promote relaxation. These behaviors can

reduce cortisol levels, increase mood, and promote metabolic balance.

3. Consistent Physical Task: Exercise is an excellent stress absorber and can help prevent the detrimental effects of prolonged stress on metabolism. Regular physical activity, such as aerobic exercise, weight training, or yoga, can help to lower hormones associated with stress, improve mood, and boost metabolic function.

4. Healthy Coping methods: Practicing healthy coping methods will help you manage stress and avoid emotional eating and other harmful behaviors. This might involve spending time with family and friends, doing hobbies, setting boundaries, requesting help from others, or engaging in self-care activities.

Aim for a healthy way of life that includes self-care, leisure, and hobbies that offer you joy and fulfillment. Taking pauses, scheduling leisure, and finding methods to relax can all help decrease stress and improve metabolic health.

7.1.2 Sleep promotes metabolic balance

1. Hormonal Controls: Adequate sleep is necessary for controlling hormones associated with hunger regulation, digestion, and energy balance. Sleep deprivation alters the hormonal equilibrium of hormones such as leptin and ghrelin, resulting in increased appetite, cravings, and changes in energy expenditure.

2. Restoration Procedures: While sleeping, the body performs vital restorative functions such as tissue repair, muscular development, and hormone control. Adequate sleep facilitates these processes, improves cellular repair, and aids in metabolic balance.

3. Sleep regulates the amount of sugar in the blood and insulin sensitivity. Poor sleep can affect the breakdown of glucose, raise insulin sensitivity, and

raise the risk of metabolic diseases including type 2 diabetes as well as obesity.

4. Cognitive Functionality: Proper sleep is necessary for cognitive function, retention of memories, and capacity to make decisions. Lack of sleep can impair cognitive function, raise stress, and have a detrimental influence on dietary decisions and eating habits.

5. Sleep Hygiene Practices:Developing appropriate sleep hygiene habits can help enhance sleep quality and metabolic balance. This includes sticking to a regular sleeping pattern, developing a calming evening ritual, optimizing the sleep environment (dark, quiet, and comfy), minimizing time spent on screens before bed, and preventing caffeine and heavy meals prior to bedtime.

To summarize, emphasizing stress management and excellent sleep is critical to preserving metabolic balance, improving overall health, and attaining weight control objectives. By combining thoughtful practices, healthy coping methods, regular physical exercise, and excellent sleeping routines into your everyday life, you may boost your metabolism and improve your overall health.

Chapter 8
Tracking Progress and Celebrating Success

8.0 Journaling Your Metabolism Makeover Journey

Journaling your metabolic makeover journey may be a successful method for self-examination tracking progress, and remaining inspired along the road. Here's how to keep a detailed log of your metabolic transformation journey:

1. Set Clear Intentions: Begin by establishing clear goals for your metabolic transformation quest. Define your goals, motives, and desired results. What are you hoping to accomplish with this process? Put down your goals in your diary so they might act as a beacon of inspiration for you on your path.

2. Record Your Starting place: Begin your notebook by recording your starting place. Record pertinent information including your present weight and evaluations, body structure, fitness level, dietary routine, sleeping habits, level of stress, and overall health. This baseline will be used as a starting point for measuring progress over time.

3. Develop a Journaling habit: Develop a consistent journaling habit which works for you. Set aside specific time each week or day to ponder on your encounters, ideas, feelings, and achievements. Find a time that works best for you to spend time with your journal, either it's in the early hours, before bed, or at a peaceful period in the day.

4. Reflect on Your objectives: Take some time to consider your metabolic makeover objectives and aspirations. Write about what motivated you to go on this trip, what you intend to accomplish, and why it is important to you. To maintain

concentration and motivation, revisit your goals on a frequent basis.

5. Monitor Daily behaviors: Keep a log of your daily behaviors for nutrition, physical activity, rest, coping with stress, and self-care. Keep track of your dietary and drinking habits, workout routine, sleeping hours and excellence, levels of stress, and any other important lifestyle factors. Be honest and nonjudgmental about your observations.

6. Assess Emotions and Reactions: Journaling provides a safe environment to examine your feelings, ideas, and triggers connected to nutrition, physical activity, and overall well-being. Write about your accomplishments, problems, desires, temptations, wins, challenges, and any emotions you experience along the journey. Recognize trends and probable causes for emotional snacking or stress.

7. Celebrate your successes, no matter how minor. Recognize and appreciate your accomplishments,

milestones, and triumphs along the path. Write about successful events, personal growth, and good changes that have occurred as a consequence of your efforts.

8. Gain knowledge from Setbacks: View setbacks as lessons to be learned rather than failures. When confronted with a difficulty or failure, use your notebook to ponder on what occurred, what you have acquired, and how you may go ahead. Write about ways for conquering challenges and remaining courageous in the midst of hardship.

9. Show Gratitude: Develop a gratitude mindset by writing about what you're thankful for in your life, such as your body, well-being, social life, experiences, and accomplishments. Expressing appreciation can help you change your perspective, improve your mood, and build resilience.

10. Envisage Success: Use your notebook to envisage your success and the future you want. Write about your desires, goals, and the kind of life

you want for yourself. Visualize yourself reaching your objectives, living a full and meaningful life, and being the best form of you.

11. Evaluate and Reflect: Review the journal entries on a regular basis to keep track of your progress, find trends, and get insights into your routines and actions. Reflect on your trip, noting what works well and what aspects may need to be adjusted or refined. Apply this reflection to guide your next moves and keep going forward with your metabolic transformation.

Your journal can be a helpful companion on your journey to long-lasting health and vitality. By implementing these record keeping policies into your metabolism makeover, you can gain insightful knowledge, be responsible to your targets, and develop a more profound awareness of your attention and your connection with food, exercise, and your general health.

8.1 Setting Goals for Continued Health and Fitness

Setting objectives for ongoing health and fitness is critical for keeping motivated, engaged, and committed to progress toward your long-term well-being. Here's how to develop useful goals for your continuing journey:

1. Focus on Your Core Principles and Priorities: Begin by examining your beliefs, your priorities, and what is most important to you when it comes to of wellness and physical fitness. Consider what inspires you, what provides you joy, and your long-term goals. Your objectives should be consistent with your basic principles and personal desires.

2. Establish SMART goals, or specific, measurable, achievable, relevant, and time-bound objectives: Establish SMART objectives, which stand for precise, measurable, achievable, relevant, and time-bound. Instead of aiming for broad or nebulous

objectives, make sure your goals are precise, attainable, and time-bound. Rather than stating "I aim to get myself in shape," for instance, you may make a target like "I will be running a 5K race within 3 months."

3. Divide Your Objectives: Divide more ambitious objectives into smaller, more doable deadlines or stages of action. This helps you monitor your progress more efficiently and lessens the overwhelming nature of your goals. For example, divide your six-month weight reduction goal of twenty pounds into small monthly or weekly goals.

4. Prioritize Behavior-Based Goals: Give priority to behavior-based goals that are under your control rather than only outcome-based ones (such as achieving a specific weight loss target). This might include objectives for stress reduction (e.g., regular meditation practice), sleep (e.g., obtaining 7 hours of sleep each night), workout (e.g., working out at

least three times a week), or diet (e.g., eating more veggies).

5. Develop Simultaneously Short-term and long-term success: To give your fitness and health journey direction and structure, set goals for the short and long term. While long-term objectives offer a feeling of purpose and a future vision, short-term targets can help you maintain motivation and momentum.

6. Create Goals Customized and Flexible: Customize your goals to meet your own requirements, tastes, and circumstances. What works for another person may not be effective for you, so set objectives that are significant and applicable to your own circumstances. Be willing to change your goals in response to shifting priorities, obstacles, or opportunities.

7. Incorporate Several Aspects of Health and Exercise:Approach goal planning holistically, taking into account your physical health, nutrition,

mental wellness, how well you sleep, dealing with stress, and general lifestyle habits. Balancing objectives in all of these areas can result in long-term benefits in your physical and mental wellness.

8. Track Development and Celebrate Achievements:Keep track of your progress and successes on a regular basis. Journals, apps, and progress charts may help you record your accomplishments, manage your activities, and stay responsible to your goals. Celebrate milestones and victories, no matter how minor, to boost positive behavior and keep motivation high.

9. Request Assistance and Accountability: Share your objectives with friends, family, or a supportive group to get encouragement, accountability, and direction. Establishing a support system may help you maintain your drive, overcome barriers, and handle problems as they arise.

10. Evaluate and Modify Your Goals as Needed: Review your goals from time to time to see how

you're doing, pinpoint areas that need work, and make any necessary revisions. Be adaptable and ready to modify your objectives in response to new information learned on your trip, feedback, or changing circumstances.

You may make a plan for success and give yourself the tools you need to have a full, active life by creating meaningful, attainable, and individualized objectives for your ongoing fitness and well-being.

Chapter 9
Conclusion
Your Metabolism Makeover

9.0 Reflecting on Your Transformation

Reflecting on your change during a metabolic makeover experience is a beneficial habit that helps you to celebrate your accomplishments, gather insights, and find areas for improvement.

Here are some useful ways to reflect on your transformation:

1. Acknowledge Your Achievements: Begin by recognizing and praising your accomplishments along the road. Take time to acknowledge your progress, no matter how modest.

2. Celebrate milestones wins, and moments of achievement that represent good improvements in

your wellness, dietary habits, and overall well-being.

3. Review your goals: Review the targets you outlined at the start of your metabolic transformation journey. Consider the extent to which you've advanced and whether you've accomplished progress toward your early goals. Identify objectives you've accomplished and those that require revision or modification based on your knowledge and experiences you've obtained along the way.

4. Evaluate Physical Modifications: Consider any physical modifications you've seen during your metabolic transformation journey. This may involve changes in weight, composition of the body, metrics, level of fitness, energy levels, or general look. Examine how your body behaves and operates different as outcome of your activities.

5. Investigate Behavioral Shifts: Think about any alterations in your behaviors, routines, and ways of

life since starting your metabolic makeover. Consider the new behaviors you've developed, the old habits you've abandoned, and the obstacles you've faced along the way. Consider how your everyday habits, decisions, and actions have developed to benefit your physical and mental well-being.

6. Evaluate Emotional and Psychological Shifts: Consider any emotions or mental changes you've had during your metabolic transformation journey. Observe changes in your mood, mentality, confidence, self-esteem, and general emotional well-being. Consider how your connection with nourishment, physical activity, and self-care has changed over time.

7. Identify Lessons learnt: Think about the lessons you've learnt during your metabolic transformation journey. Consider what has worked best for you, what problems you've encountered, and what you've learned about oneself, your physical appearance,

and your health. Identify useful lessons learnt that you can apply in the future.

8. Express Gratitude: Develop a grateful mindset by showing appreciation for your trip and development. Take a time to thank everyone who has helped you with your progress. Be grateful for your present of wellness and good health.

9. Set New intents: Use your thoughts to help shape new intents and objectives for the next stage of your metabolic transformation journey. Consider what improvements you want to keep selecting what areas you want to put your energies on next, and your long-term health and well-being goals.

Finally, enjoy your change and who you've achieved as a consequence of your metabolic makeover adventure. Accept the road of self-discovery, development, and change, knowing that each step you've made brings you closer to a happier, healthier, and more vibrant existence.

Spending the time to reflect on your change throughout the metabolism makeover journey may provide you with useful insights, expand your awareness of yourself, and foster thankfulness for the progress you've accomplished. Use this contemplation as a starting point for future development, progress, and wellness in all aspects of your life.

9.1 Embracing a Healthier, Energetic, and Fitter You!

Cultivating a healthier, more energetic, and stronger version of yourself involves learning about oneself, self-care, and personal development. It entails making intentional decisions that consider your mental, emotional, and physical wellness, as well as cultivating a positive connection within oneself and your body. Here are some methods for adopting a healthier, more energized, and fitter self.

1. Nourish Your Body: Eat healthy meals that will help you achieve your health, energy, and fitness objectives. Consume a balanced diet high in veggies, fruits, lean proteins, grains that are whole, and healthy fats. Pay attention to your body's fullness and hunger cues, and use eating with consciousness to savor and appreciate your meals.

2. Remain Active: Include regular physical exercise in your daily schedule to enhance your fitness, increase energy, and improve general well-being. Find activities that you love, such as walking, biking, swimming, running, dancing, yoga, or strengthening exercises, and include movement into your daily routine.

3. Value Sleeping: Consider sleep a priority by sticking to a regular sleep schedule, developing a soothing nighttime ritual, and improving your sleep environment. Aim for seven to nine hours of good sleep every night to promote physical recuperation, mental clarity, and metabolic health.

4. Minimize Stress:To reduce stress and promote relaxation, use stress management strategies that include meditation, breathing techniques such as yoga, and journaling. Employ self-care activities that allow you to relax, refuel, and build inner calm in the face of life's obstacles.

5. Remain Hydrated: Drink enough of water during the day to keep your body hydrated and functioning properly. Carry a water container that is reusable with you and drink water on a regular basis to avoid dehydration, increase your level of energy, and maintain general health.

6. Employ self-compassion to achieve a better, more active, and fitter lifestyle. Celebrate your accomplishments, accept your flaws, and treat yourselves with the same level of love and understanding that you would give to a friend.

7. Set reasonable and achievable objectivesthat are consistent with your beliefs, priorities, and lifestyle. Break down huge goals into smaller, more

manageable tasks, and celebrate each accomplishment along the way. Focus on progress instead of excellence, and be gentle with yourself while working.

8. Surrounding Yourself with Assistance: Surround yourself with an encouraging circle of acquaintances, close relatives, or like-minded people who will motivate and support you on your path to improved health. Look for accountability partners, exercise pals, or online groups who share your aims and beliefs.

9. Embrace Moderation: Aim for balance in all aspects of your life, such as diet, physical activity, job, relationships, and leisure. Listen to your body, respect your limits, and prioritize things that give you joy, achievement, and a renewed sense of purpose.

10. Appreciate Your Achievements: Take time to acknowledge your accomplishments, no matter how minor. Recognize your accomplishments, ponder on

the way you've come, and be grateful for the chance to live a healthier, more energetic, and fitter lifestyle.

By accepting and implementing these ideas into your everyday life, you may become a healthier, more vibrant, and stronger version of yourself, exuding energy, strength, and well-being. Remember that change is a journey, and each action you take to greater health is a stride toward a more promising and vibrant future.

www.ingramcontent.com/pod-product-compliance
Lightning Source LLC
Chambersburg PA
CBHW050811250726
48653CB00006B/2164